My Brother, MPS, and Me!

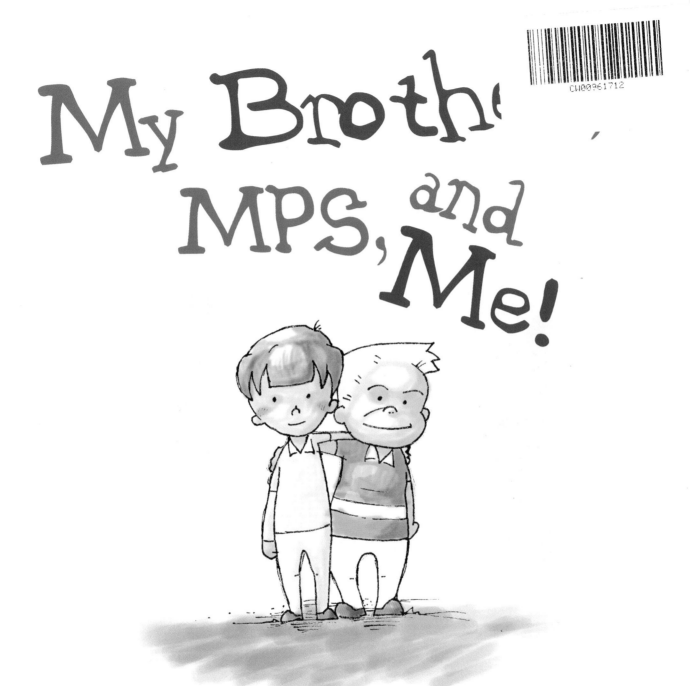

Written by Dawn A. Laney and Stephanie R. Cagle

Illustrated by Michael J. Johnson

ISBN: 1463698909
ISBN 13: 9781463698904

In Memory of Dr. Paul M. Fernhoff who worked tirelessly throughout his career to help patients, family members, and medical professionals understand complex genetic conditions like the MPSs.

My name is Greg.
My brother Daniel is my best
friend.

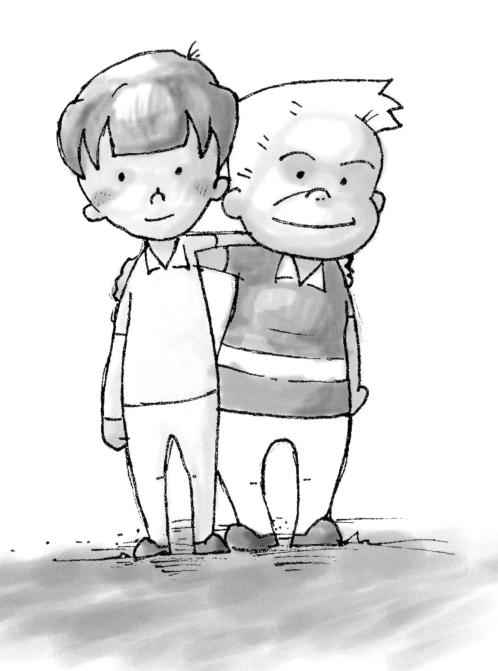

We play games.

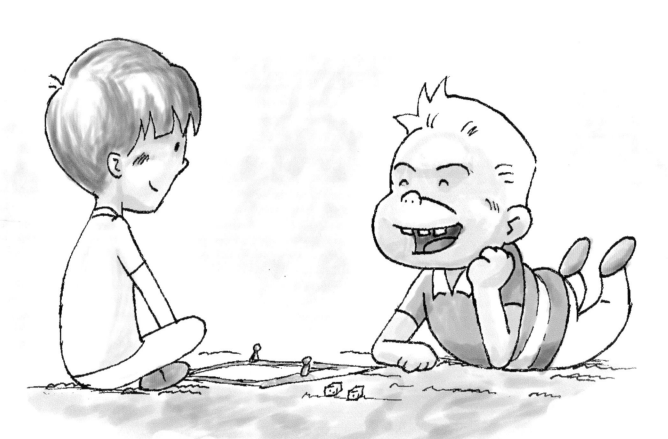

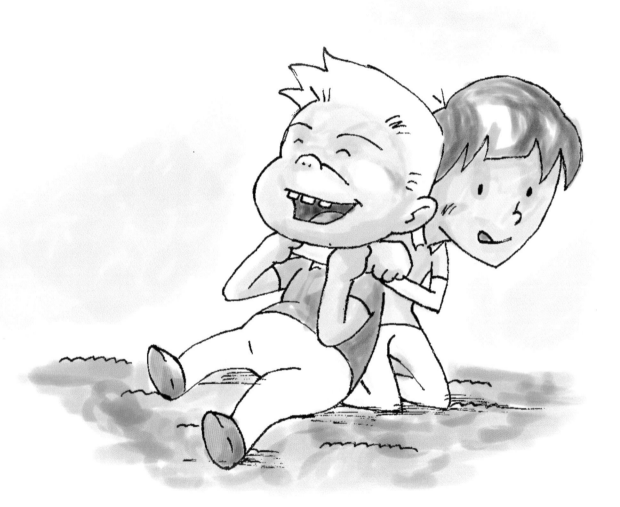

We swim.

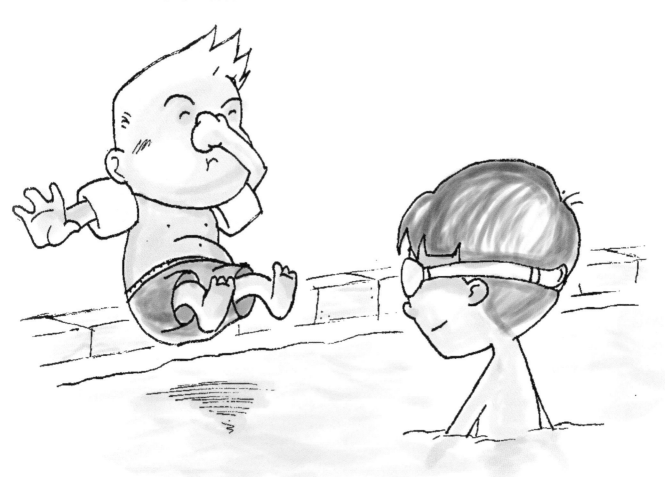

We paint.

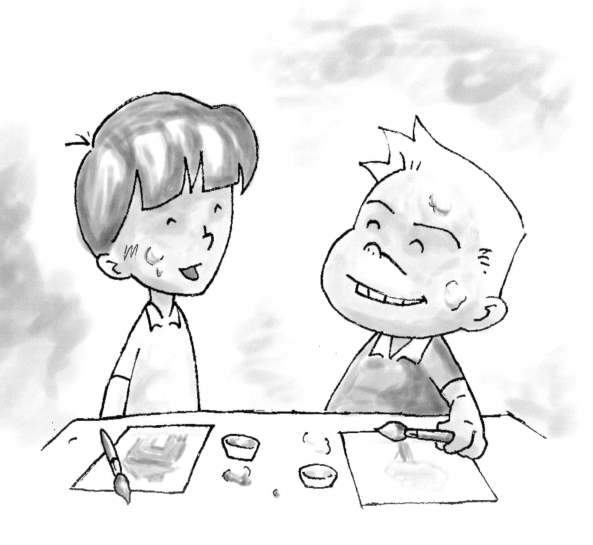

We do magic tricks.

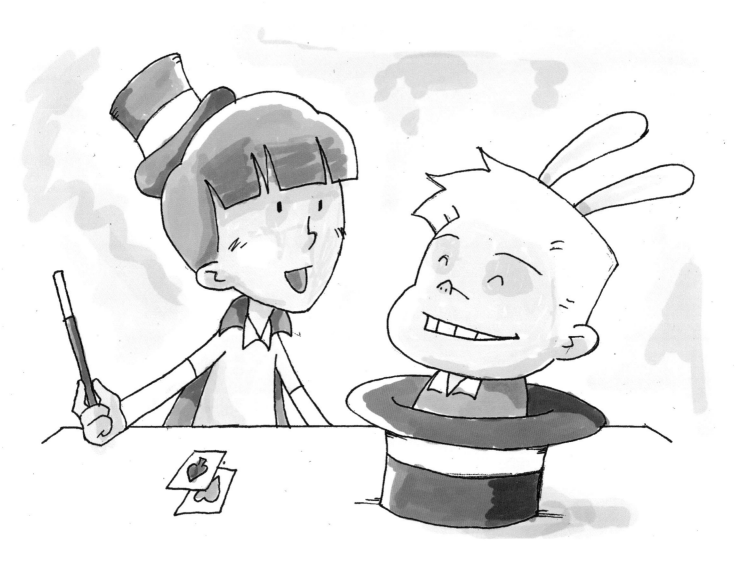

We do our chores together.

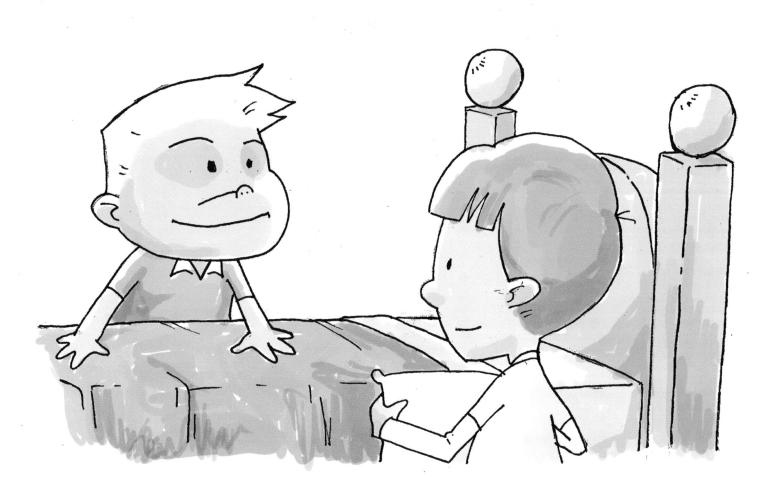

We like the same things...mostly.
Sometimes we fight...

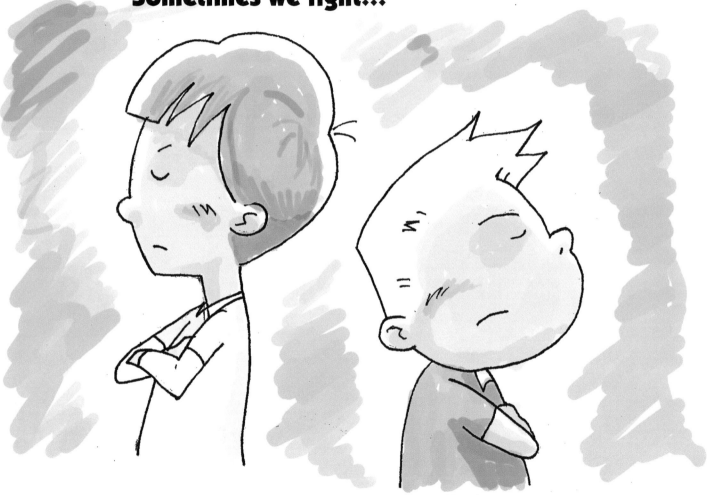

but we always make up.

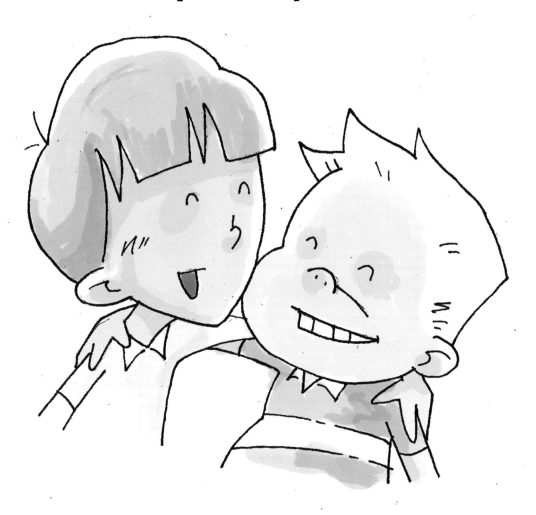

Some days, Daniel is extra tired, his hands are too stiff, or his body hurts so we have Quiet day.

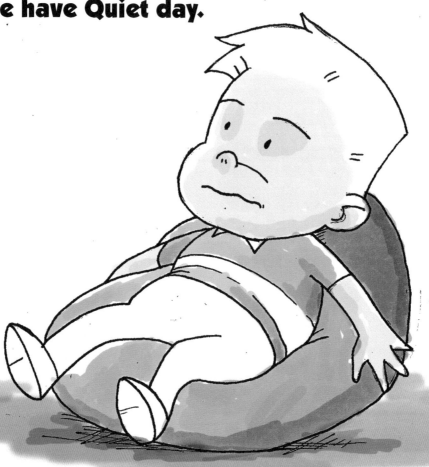

On Quiet day we may watch movies, play video games, or read books.

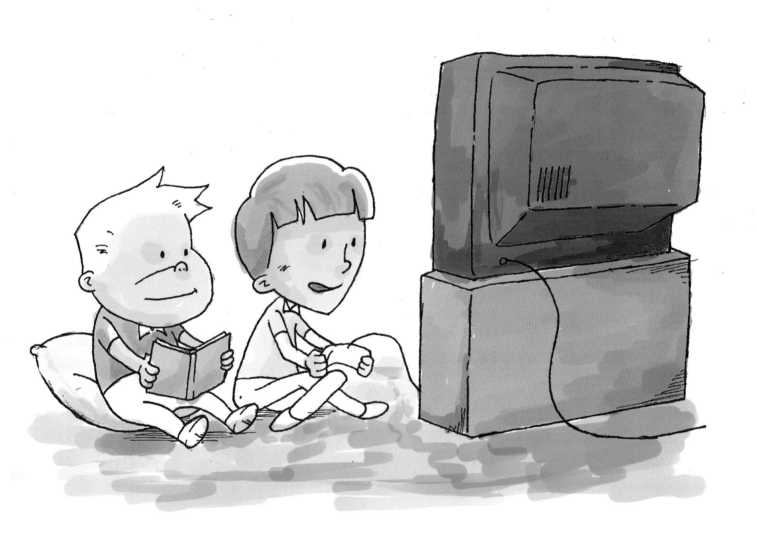

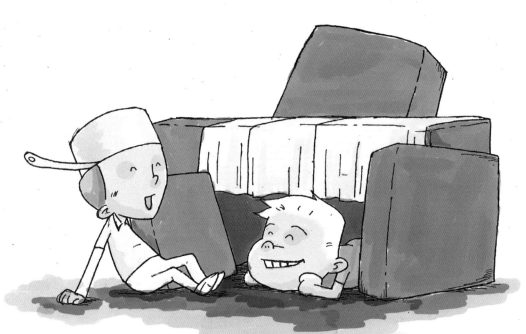

We might build a couch fort and be lazy guards.

Sometimes he's the audience and I'm the funny show.

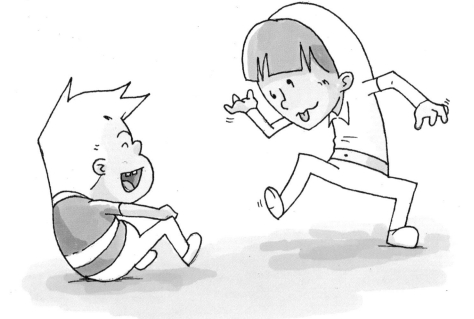

There is one big thing that my brother and I don't do together...

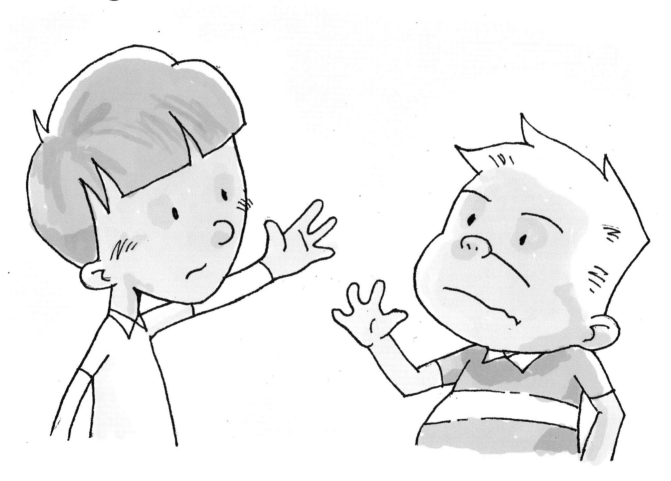

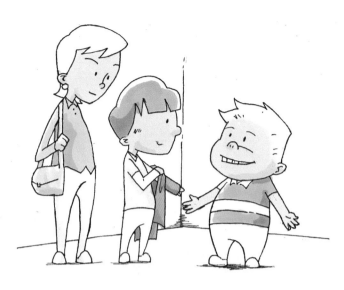

Once a week Daniel goes to a special place called an infusion center and gets his medicine. I think he's lucky because he gets out of school early AND gets to play video games for 4 HOURS!

If there is no school, I go with him.

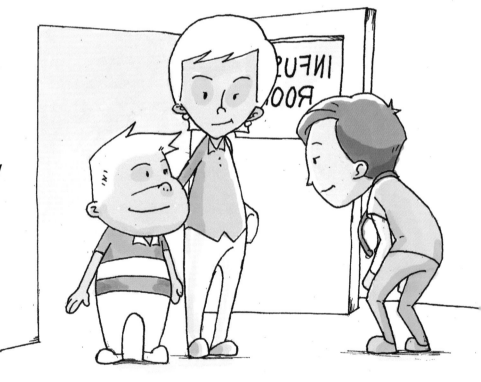

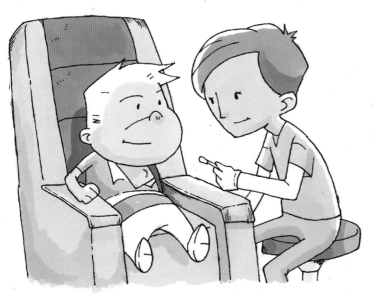

First, they put the no hurt cream on his special port bump where they give the medicine.

Then the nice nurse, Trudi, sticks the magic straw called a catheter into his port.

It doesn't hurt him a bit, but it is important for him to keep still like a statue while she's doing it.

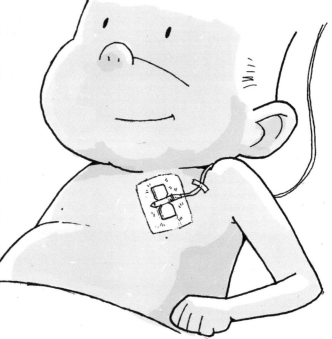

The straw is hooked to a tube and his little bag of medicine. A little machine moves the medicine from the bag, through the tube and straw, and into Daniel.

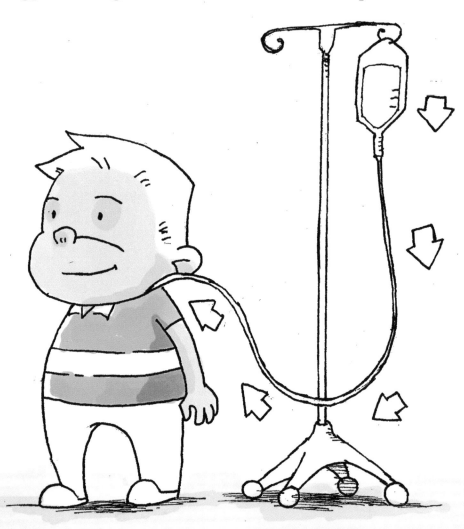

Once the machine is all hooked up, we play video games, watch movies, and eat snacks, all while my brother is getting his medicine!

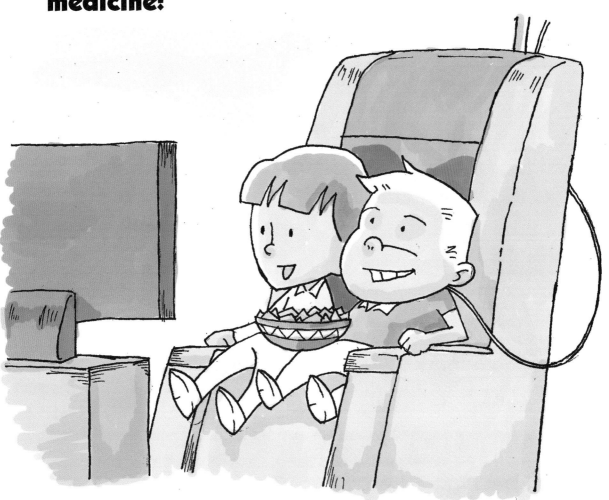

Every once in a while Trudi interrupts our games to check on things or the genetic counselor and doctor come to ask questions. They also ask if we have any questions or need to talk about anything. Infusions are fun; I wish I could go more!

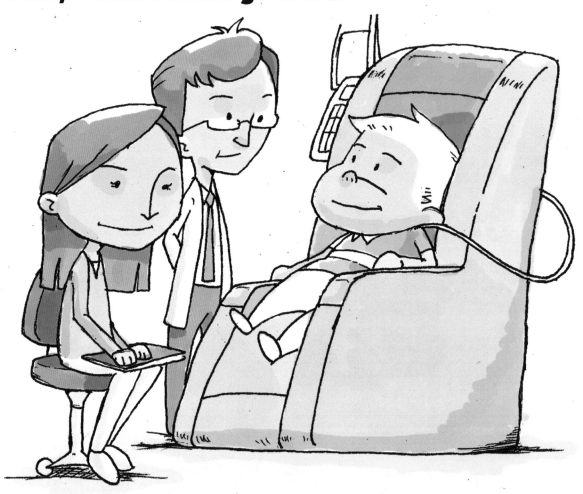

Being a brother is not all fun and games though. Sometimes I'm scared because my brother gets sicker than me from colds.

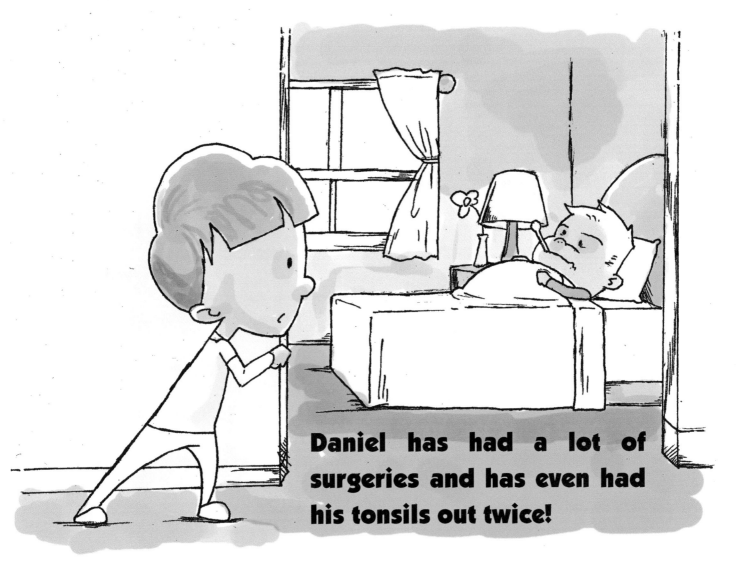

Daniel has had a lot of surgeries and has even had his tonsils out twice!

My mom said it is because he has Mucopolysaccharidosis or MPS and it makes it harder for his body to fight germs. It's also why his arms, legs, and back don't straighten out like mine.

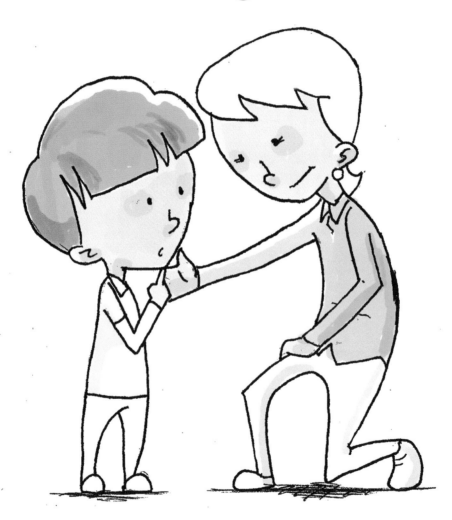

Because of MPS Daniel has to go to more doctors than me and have lots of different pictures taken of his organs and bones. He told me some of the pictures are taken by big machines that look like spaceships!

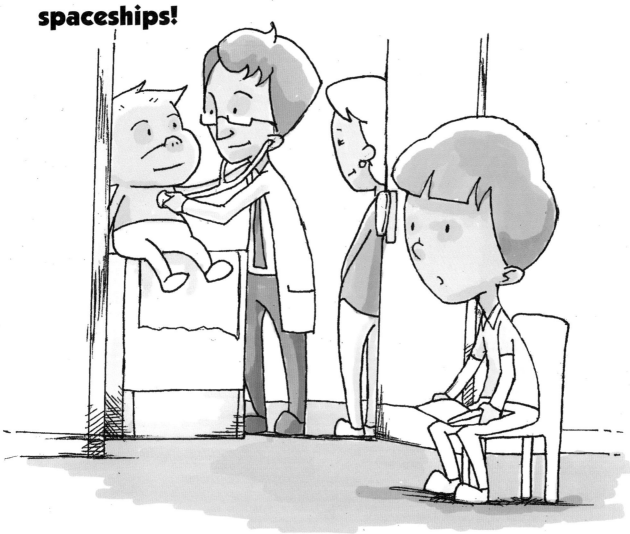

MPS happens because one of the chemicals that my brother's body needs to work is broken and some gunk has built up in his body.

The gunk makes his tonsils big, his bones short, his elbows stiff, his hands hurt, and his heart valves leaky.

The chemical in my body is working so that is why I don't have MPS too.

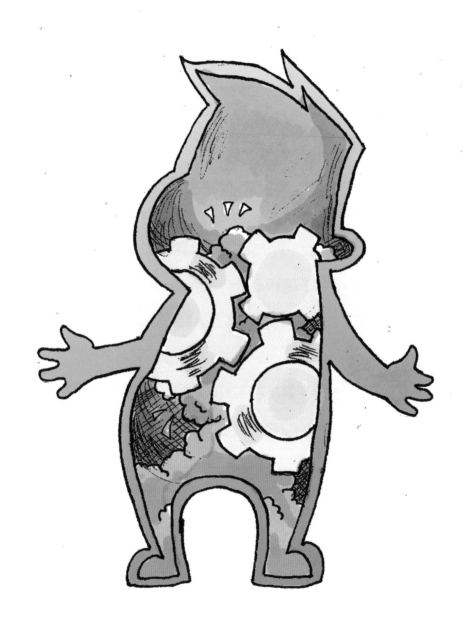

It is hard to understand, but it helps to think of it like our bodies are bathtubs. In order to keep our bathtubs clean and ready for baths, we need a drain that works. My brother's bathtub has a clogged drain and so the water overflows the bathtub, making a mess. Just like the bathtub, his body is building up gunk and that makes him get sick easily. He is given the medicine every week at the infusion center because it gets rid of some of the gunk in his body.

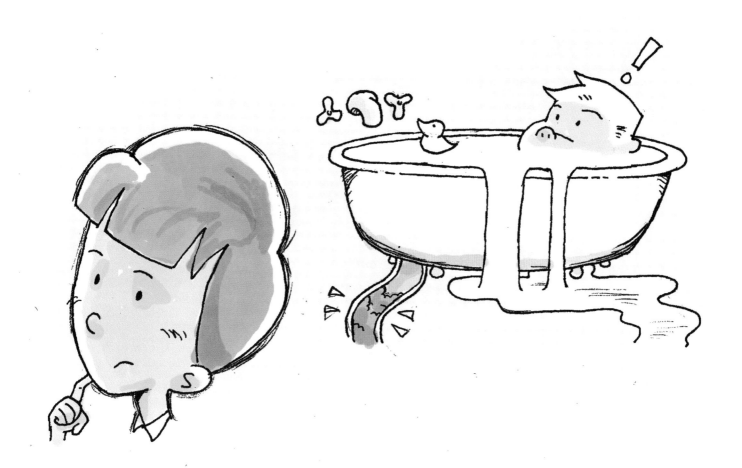

I know though, that my brother is not the only one with MPS.

Once a year we have a meeting with other MPS kids and their families.

We eat spaghetti and play while our parents talk to one another and listen to speakers.

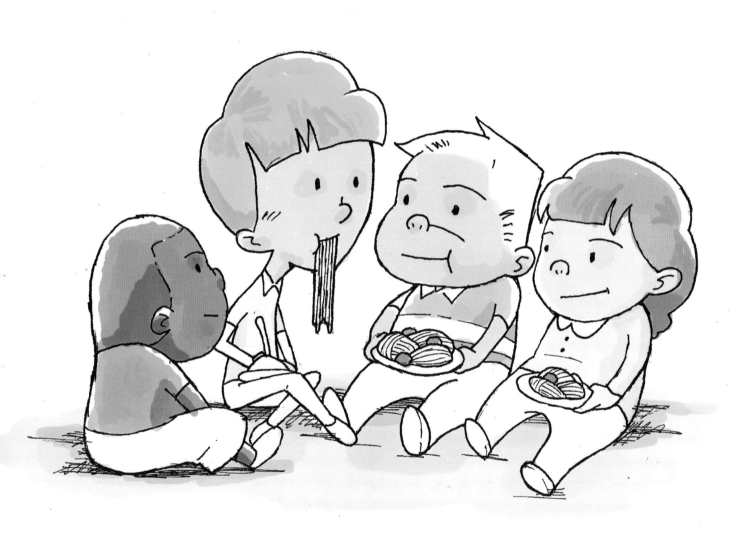

Not every kid with MPS is just like Daniel.
Some kids run like the wind, while some kids
are in wheelchairs.

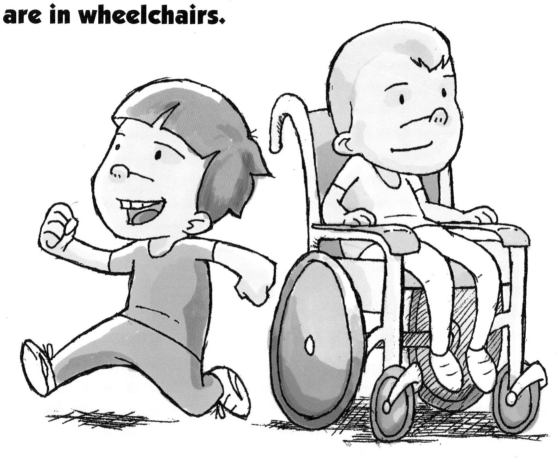

Some kids don't talk much, while others talk a lot.

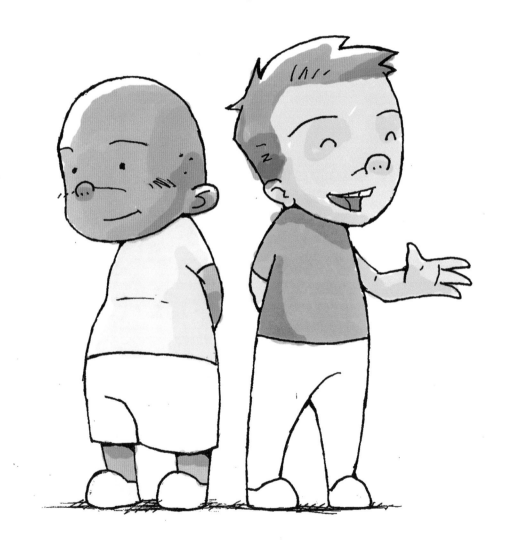

Some kids have a tube in their throat to help them breathe, and others don't.

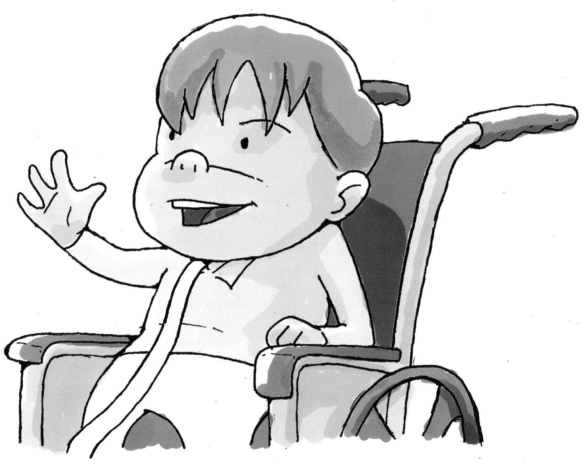

Some kids don't get medicine because they had a special treatment when they were little called a transplant.

Whatever their differences, they all are fun to play with at the meeting.

Also it's nice to know that there are other MPS families like ours.

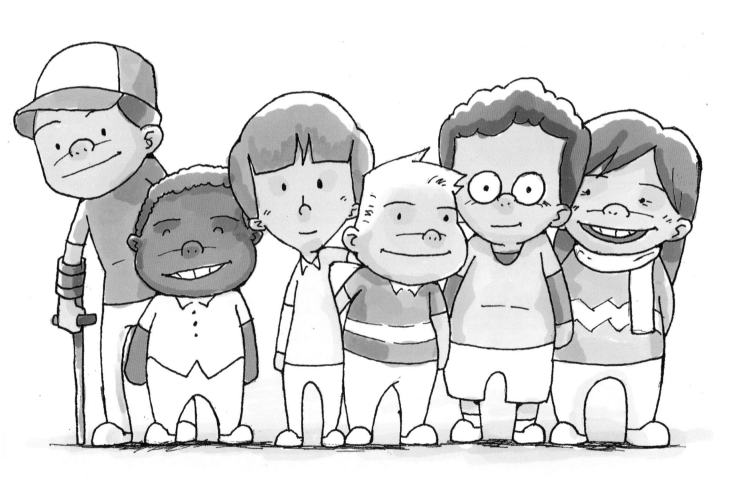

Lots of kids don't understand why my brother is different from them because they have never met someone with MPS before.

So I tell them about it and before long everyone is playing together and having fun.

We are all different from each other anyway.

I will always love Daniel no matter what.

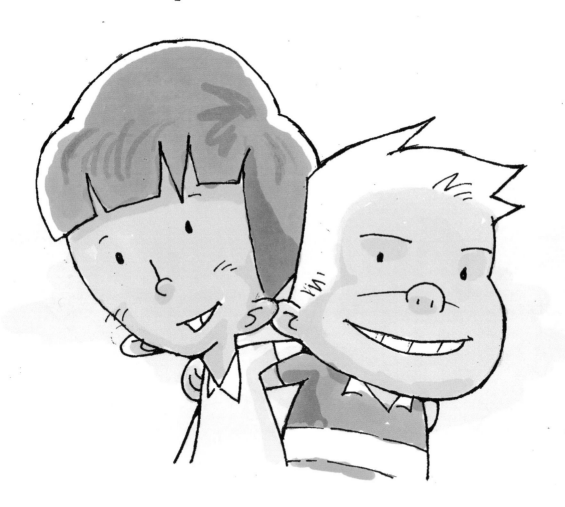

My brother is my best friend AND he has MPS.

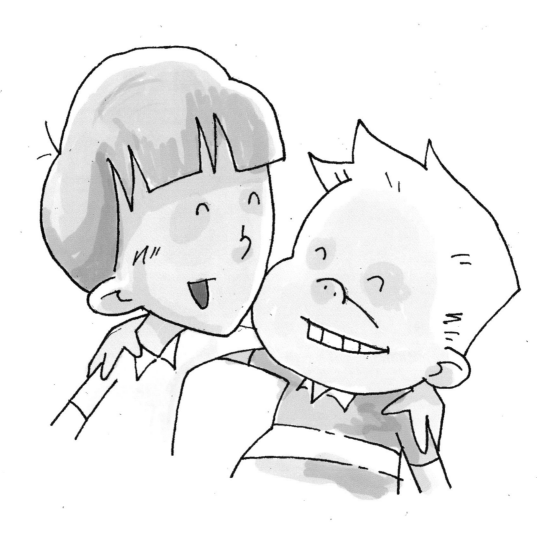

Dawn Laney and Stephanie Cagle are genetic counselors and research coordinators at the Emory Lysosomal Storage Disease Center (LSDC). They work closely with families affected by lysosomal storage diseases such as the Mucopolysaccharidoses (MPSs) and also will always love their brothers (and sister) no matter what.

Michael Johnson is an illustrator and graphic artist living in the Atlanta, GA area. He has first-hand knowledge of the impact of lysosomal storage diseases (LSDs) on families as he is affected by another LSD, Fabry disease.

Emory's Lysosomal Storage Disease Center in Atlanta, GA provides diagnosis, evaluation, management, and treatment services for patients from all over the United States.

The Center is devoted to remaining on the cutting edge of research and treatment by providing comprehensive and compassionate care for all of our patients affected by lysosomal storage diseases such as the MPS conditions.

To speak with a member of our LSD team, call 404-778-8565 or 800-200-1524. You can also visit our website at http://genetics.emory.edu/LSD

Note:

Our brothers' story was developed to help explain the MPS (or Mucopolysaccharidoses) conditions and their treatment from the perspective of a young child. Children affected by an MPS condition may have different symptoms and therapies than those described in this book. The MPS conditions are a group of inherited metabolic disorders caused by the absence or malfunction of a specific chemical or enzyme needed to break down molecules called glycosaminoglycans (or GAGs). GAGs are chains of carbohydrates in each of our cells that help build bone, cartilage, tendons, corneas, skin and connective tissue. When the GAGs are not broken down, they are stored throughout the body within the cell's lysosomes. The result is progressive cellular damage that affects appearance, physical abilities, and organ and system functioning. There are 8 different types of MPS conditions with different symptoms and available treatments. All of the conditions are progressive multisystem disorders with features ranging over a continuum from mild to severe.

The top 10 clues that tell a parent that their child may have MPS are:

Frequent ear infections	Short stature
Noisy breathing	Distinguished facial features
Stiff joints	Heart valve problems
Abnormal spine	Cloudy corneas (not in all forms of MPS)
Inguinal (in the groin) and/or Umbilical (belly button) hernias	Enlarged tonsils and adenoids

This book was published with the assistance of educational grants from Genzyme Corporation and Shire Human Genetic Therapies, Inc.

For more information about the symptoms or treatment of MPS conditions, please contact the Emory Lysosomal Storage Disease Center at 800-200-1524 or visit our website at
http://genetics.emory.edu/LSD

Additional resources can be found at the
National MPS Society website at:
http://www.mpssociety.org/

Printed in Great Britain
by Amazon.co.uk, Ltd.,
Marston Gate.